A Short Guide To
Hacking Your
Nervous System
For Better Performance
And Less Stress

ROB HARTMAN

Disclaimer: The content presented in this book is meant for educational purposes only. The purchaser of this book understands that the author is not a medical professional, and the information contained within this book is not intended to replace medical advice or meant to be relied upon to treat, cure, or prevent any disease, illness, or medical condition. It is understood that you will seek full medical clearance by a licensed physician before making any changes mentioned in this book. The author claims no responsibility to any person or entity for any liability, loss, or damage caused or alleged to be caused directly or indirectly as a result of the use, application, or interpretation of the material in this book. The purchase of this book does not establish a client-practitioner or patient-doctor relationship between the purchaser and the author.

Affiliate disclaimer: The author may have an affiliate relationship with some of the products or services that are recommended in this document. Stress Resilience Institute may earn affiliate income if you purchase these products or services through the links in this book, while the prices remain the same for you. This does not affect our choices as these are the products and services that we personally use and recommend to our clients, whether or not an affiliate relationship is possible.

Any inquiries or comments can be sent to robert.hartman@gmail.com

Testimonials For My Corporate & Personal Training Classes

This was the most relaxed I've felt in months. It wasn't laborious, just bliss.
— D. Kagan

I came in with very little knowledge of the

parasympathetic nervous system. At the end of the class, I had an understanding of what stress does to my body and how it holds on to it. I went away feeling relaxed, euphoric, and eager to practice these techniques.
— Wade, Wounded Operation Iraqi Freedom

Really cool stuff. I'm usually cynical about

this sort of thing, but really enjoyed it.
— G. Kemper

A great class - easy to follow and a great

break from a hectic work week!
— A. Dewey

Rob's insight and teaching have opened my

eyes to not only the power of the human body
and the dangers of being in a chronic state of
high stress, but also our ability to down-
regulate and change that through a variety of
breathing and release methods. This is exactly
what I have needed for so long I will definitely
be back for more.
— Ellen, workshop participant and travel
consultant

DEDICATION

This book is dedicated to my self
and my nervous system.
My hope is that you'll dedicate
these practices to your self.
You are worth it.

CONTENTS

Acknowledgements

I am grateful to have many teachers. Here's a short list of those who have positively influenced this book:

David Berceli, Phd	Sri Sri Ravi Shankar
Teri Cochrane, CN	Peter Levine, Phd
Tara Brach, Phd	Raymon Grace
Sri Nisargadatta	Jonathan FitzGordon
Evan Rabinowitz, MAC	Diettrich Klinghardt, MD
Leila Zachrison, MD	Ginger Sullivan, LPC
Dennis Shackley	Liz Koch
Sherry Cupac, MSW	Bill Pullen, MS
John Douillard, DC	Wim Hof

I am grateful to have many students. Each of whom I have learned so much from. Thank you for modeling the courage and persistence to do the work.

Varun Moktan played an integral role in bringing this manuscript to life. Somehow, he was able to transform scratch notes, theories delivered at high speed on video conference, and incomprehensible handwriting into a readable book. Thank you Varun.

This book wouldn't have been possible without the help and encouragement of countless supporters and brainstorm partners including: Rob H, Travis Rumsey, Ron, Anita, David, Trent, Carol, Maria, Carolyn, my bros from Mankind, Michael, Michelle, Greg, Ana, DC Toastmasters, and many others.

Thank you to Bobby Ross from District Photographics for the photos.

Intro

If you would have told me in my 20s that I'd go hang out with neuroscientists, Native American shamans, and Yogi Monks, I would have told you that you were crazy. But that's exactly what I did. In 2009, my life hit a breaking point and I crashed. I left my job and began a quest to find ancient and advanced methods to hack the nervous system into deep states of relaxation. From the mountains of India where I meditated with yogis and gurus to working with Native American shamans, I have learned and borrowed so many techniques.

Complex systems have always fascinated me. In high school, I would spend hours at the junk yard learning how to put cars together and take them apart. At some point, that fascination transitioned to computers. In 1993, I got my first computer and quickly started learning how to break it.

It was a 486 DX2 66 Mhz. It had a turbo button, which was a critical feature. Everyone in the military school hall was jealous of the speed of my computer. It had turbo mode! Turbo mode allowed me to play games at blazing speed and get that rush. I craved the hit of adrenaline while sitting at the computer.

But turning the turbo off was vital at certain points. Some games were unplayable with it. If you didn't turn off turbo, everything would happen too fast. The voices and special effects would be unrecognizable.

Throughout my 20s, I lived life in that turbo mode. I had a fast-paced life of great work gigs, travel, long hours, and lots of successes. It was great... I climbed a ladder toward the image of success.

But there was a serious problem... I was stuck in turbo mode. Sleep was bad. I had constant anxiety or depression. I was burning out daily. I would have days of 6-shot cappuccinos, energy drinks until 4 pm, and then switch to wine and whiskey to calm down. A pack and a half of cigarettes and Xanax barely slowed me down. Friends would say, "just relax." I had no idea how. I had no experience in relaxing and enjoying the small things. I was stuck in a mode of doing and not being. I was stuck in turbo mode. It's common but unnatural.

The handful of prescriptions wasn't working. My doctor warned that I wouldn't live another 10 years.

I had to do something different... A quote rang in my head for days, "If you always do what you've always done, you'll always get what you've always gotten." I needed something different – and so the journey to find a totally new way of living began.

I wrote this book to not only shed light on some of the research and findings of how we can modulate our autonomic nervous system, but also as a guide book to help you realize a healthier life. These are the techniques, mindsets, and ideas that I've collected and refined through years of hardship and pain. These are the culmination of seven years of agony and ecstasy from my travels across the world. And finally, these are the gems of my own journey –

insights I wish someone had told me when times were dark.

I still have stress in my life. But now I have a set of tools to help reduce it.

The goal isn't to eliminate stress. The goal is to make you more powerful and the stress non-sticky – in essence, to make you able to bounce back from stress… to be resilient.

I hope this book will be a companion in your journey for relaxation and peace of mind.

Chapter 1: Intro to the Autonomic Nervous System

The autonomic nervous system (ANS) is the key system of the body that handles stress. Think of it as the acceleration/deceleration system of your body. It has two modes: on and go, or off and slow.

When you're in the car and want to go faster, you hit the "gas pedal." In your body, that's the fight-flight part that's also called the sympathetic nervous system or "on/go." If you want your car to slow down, then you hit the brake pedal. In your body, the braking system is called the parasympathetic nervous system or "off/slow."

Some people at first have no interest in slowing down. I get it. For years, I didn't want to slow down. The problem is that things that don't slow down eventually burn up or crash.

Here are some signs that your braking system (or parasympathetic nervous system) could be improved:

- You have problems sleeping
- You are irritable or cranky
- You often feel anxiety
- You are depressed

(For any medical condition, please go see a qualified medical professional and use this book as a guide to understand what's going on within your body.)

At every moment, your ANS is adjusting your heart rate, breathing rate, digestion, sexual response, and many intricate facets of the body to respond or react to your perception of how the current moment is. For example, if you're running from a tiger, the ANS will shift the focus to survival. Blood and resources will flow toward the large muscles required for fighting or running. You'll go into turbo mode. Now, if you're running from a tiger, this might not seem like a big deal because, well, you're *running from a tiger*. But it's important... This turbo will shift the focus away from digestion and reproduction. You'll sleep worse and be irritable.

In the modern world, we hopefully never have to run from a tiger. But this same shift to survival happens in other situations like when we receive a threatening email or phone call. Maybe we get that text we've been dreading from our ex, or even the score on that exam we thought we bombed. Our body turns sympathetic: the muscles tense, the heart rate rises, and the brain switches to survival. Thus, our perception plays a big role in this happening of the body.

———————————

Our entire body tends to be in either survival/emergency mode dictated by the sympathetic nervous system (on/go/gas pedal mode) or in relaxation mode dictated by the parasympathetic nervous system (off/slow/brake pedal mode). When we run, fight, argue, or race around, we're not allowing the body to rest, digest, or nest properly.

———————————

To help us explore both parts of the nervous system, let´s introduce Tim.

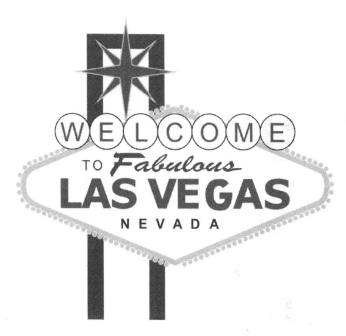

Vegas and Your Vagus

With beads of sweat rolling off his forehead, Tim looks at his watch. It's already past 2 am. As every minute passes, his heart is about to explode. He tries to tell himself to calm down and get a glass of water. As he requests one of the waiters, his hands tremble, and he gets a glimpse of his face off the reflection in a pair of glasses. He's flushed. His teeth are clenched, and he has some difficulty remembering what he just ordered.

He gasps at how much money he's lost and how dry his throat is. This was supposed to be a fun trip to hang out with executives to show them he was one of them. The dealer asks him to Hit or Stand. He's snarling: Hit. He's irritated at the dealer, and he's frustrated at the people on the other table laughing, smiling, and sharing drinks.

Most of us know Tim's story: that feeling of anxiety, panic, and stress all manifesting into frustration and rigidity. Las Vegas has excited every part of his nervous system and it cripples him. The stress, both physiological and psychological, has consequences, and Tim's body is responding. It treats the game of Blackjack in the same way it would react to an external threat. But why is Tim feeling this way? How can just losing a small hand of cards make him feel so badly?

Tim's story is a microcosm for the way our body and our ANS reacts to the world as a whole. This book is about our ways of dealing with stress. It's about techniques that I've honed throughout the years that can help to modulate our physiology. These skills help in reprogramming our nervous system, so it doesn't always revert to the primitive state of fear, anxiety, and frustration we feel in tense situations.

We need to begin with understanding how the nervous system works. But don't worry about all the jargon; I just want to give you some context about the ANS before we explore how we can modulate it, which is the focus of this book.

The promise of fun and excitement engages Tim's nervous system. He initially feels the rush of adrenaline and the pounding of his heart as he plays each hand of the game. He feels the pace of the environment around him. The glaring music, the bright lights, the flashing colors, the exchange of money, the scent of alcohol, and other external stimuli only further trigger his senses. But chronic turbo mode and exposure to stress exhausts the system. In the same way an animal cannot always be on alert for predators, humans cannot be constantly exposed to many external stimuli. Because of this, Tim's body starts to manifest burnout. He gets frustrated, and his body goes into overdrive. The threat of losing money becomes a real problem. It affects his biology as a series of hormones flushes down his body and causes him to feel stressed.

The threat of losing money and the accompanying stress activates Tim's sympathetic mode. As half of the ANS, this is the primitive system that we equate with the "fight-flight" response. This mode, gets you ready to fight or run. And it makes Tim anxious and wired.

Think of the sympathetic chain ganglia as the gas pedal. Nerve fibers that originate from Tim's spine send hormonal signals to various organs in his system. There's a rush of norepinephrine and cortisol that latches onto the receptors of various muscles and tissues, causing a variety of changes. Tim's eyes start to dilate. He sweats. His breathing gets shallow as he uses more of his chest. Other onlookers at the table might not notice his increased heart rate, but they do notice that he's panting, that his lower back has tightened, that his jaw's clenched, that his brow contracts, and that his face gets tight and contorted. He's miserable. It's the opposite of a poker face.

Tim is not relaxed, and that will lead to errors of judgment.

So if Tim's in Las Vegas and wants to be super relaxed and, as a byproduct, maintain a good poker face, then he needs to learn a few hacks. First, he must learn to empower his *vagus nerve*, and second, he must discharge any pent-up energy from his sympathetic nervous system before an important round of poker. The vagus nerve is a major component responsible for calming the body and starting a system called the parasympathetic system. Think of it as the braking mechanism. This system is all about resting, digesting, and nesting. When Tim's in this state, he's got the perfect and relaxed face. His heart rate and blood pressure are lower. To the onlooker or other people at the poker table, he looks calm, confident, and ready to play the game.

This is the opposite of the reactive and sweating version of Tim we saw earlier. This relaxed, parasympathetic mode is perfect for making bets and making love, and for being proactive rather than reactive – everything you want for a good experience in Las Vegas to last.

In fact, research has indicated that a weak vagus nerve is involved in many conditions:

- Rheumatoid arthritis sufferers have weak vagus nerve function (Waldburger et al., 2010).
- Children of depressed moms seem to have weak vagus nerves (Field & Diego, 2008).
- Parent conflict affects the respiratory sinus arrhythmia – this is the natural rhythm of the breath/heart beat connection (Moore, 2012).
- Children who stutter have weak vagal tone (Jones et al., 2014).
- ADHD is linked to low vagus nerve function (Beauchaine, 2001).

Overall, the dichotomy between sympathetic and parasympathetic can be a little confusing. Let's try to break it. The table below shows some of the signs, symptoms, and qualities of the different branches of the ANS. In future chapters, you'll learn how to influence the nervous system with breathing, body postures, and other techniques. As an example, if you'd like to digest better (or make love longer), you'd want to boost your parasympathetic function. As you can see in the table, one way to do this is to spend some time breathing deeply into the belly through the nose (aka diaphragmatic breathing).

Modes of the Autonomic Nervous System

Which Mode Are You In?	Parasympathetic "Brake Pedal"	Sympathetic "Gas Pedal"
Overall	LOVE/FAITH	FEAR
	Rest/Digest/Nest Ease – It's OK Relaxed	Emergency/Fight/Flight Disease – It's Not OK Resisting/Tense
	Joy, love, sadness	Anxiety = Fear, anger, shame
Good For:	Eating, thinking, making love, sleep	Fighting, reactivity, running
Which Nerve?	Vagus nerve	Sympathetic chain ganglia
Neurotransmitter	Acetyl-choline	Epinephrine
Asian Medicine	Yin	Yang
Lie Detector	Not sweaty	Sweaty

Machine. The lie detector is one of the best old-fashioned methods of measuring the stress level on the autonomic nervous system.	Respiration is full, long, rhythmic – The belly rises and falls	Respiration is short, uneven, into the chest
	Muscles in buttocks stay relaxed	Muscles in buttocks tense
	Heart rate decreases	Heart rate increases
	Blood pressure decreases	Blood pressure increases
Ph of body & fluids	Alkaline	Acidic
Sleep	Deep	Light
Digestion	Salivation	Dry mouth
	Good digestion	Poor digestion
Brain/ Mental	Full cortex	Brain Stem
	Strategic/Contemplative	Reactive like a reptile
	See many options	See fewer options

Face	Vision wide – Pupils sharpen	Tunnel vision – Eyes dilated
	Blush – Glow	Pale, metallic skin or flush/Beet red
	Brow relaxed	Brow furrowed
	Jaw loose – Horse sound with mouth	Jaw tight – Grinding teeth
	Tongue relaxed	Tongue on roof of mouth
Posture/ Pelvis	Back is loose, limber, pain free – Psoas loose	Back pain due to tension – Psoas tight, creating tightness in lumbar region (L4-L5)
	Expanded – Take up space – Power posing/Man spreading	Contracted – Small
	Posture expands	Posture contracts
	Chest/shoulders	Concave

	– Expanse	
Breathing	Into belly and pelvis – Diaphragmatic	Chest/Thoracic
	Nasal	Mouth
	Extended exhale	Extended inhale
Senses	Hearing expanded	Hearing focused ("tunnel hearing") or even hearing loss – We tune out
Mindset	Abundance, generous, mutual benefit	Scarce, greedy, zero sum
Inflammatory Markers	Lower	Higher
Histamine Levels	Histamine low	Histamine high
Perceived Stress Scale Score (PSS)	Low	High
Adverse Childhood	Low	High

Experiences (ACES)		
Rate of Wound Healing	Fast /Regenerative	Slow / Degenerative
Sports Recovery Time	Fast	Slow
Chance of Stuttering	Low	High
Levels of Violence & Aggression	Low	High
Aging	Age slow	Age fast
Obsession & Addiction	Low	High

Ancient cultures like the Yogis, Kung Fu Artists, and Chinese medical practitioners found interesting ways to stimulate the vagus nerve and calm the body. Some of these techniques are described in the following sections of this book. The more we can engage and grow the vagus and, consequently, the parasympathetic nervous system, the better off we'll be in handling our stress.

Let's look at this dichotomy another way.

The Rhythm of the Autonomic Nervous System (ANS)

Life includes both stress and relaxation. I've drawn a diagram (Figure 1.1) that helps to show the ebbs and flows of life. Stress can enter our lives in the form of an external threat (like a saber tooth tiger chasing after you) or the internal stress that can be manifested in anxiety, frustration, or worry. Either way, these states rev up our body. You can see the stress going "up" on the curve in Diagram 1.1. On the other hand, when we do the exercises in this book, our stress goes "down." This boosts our cognitive performance.

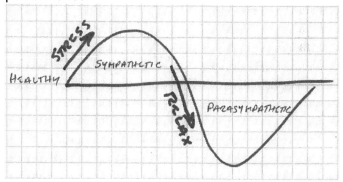

Diagram 1.1

However, this isn't as straightforward for most people. In fact, some people might constantly be stressed out. Like Tim, they could be part of a cutthroat business environment that breeds uncertainty. In fact, Tim's stress wave might look something like this:

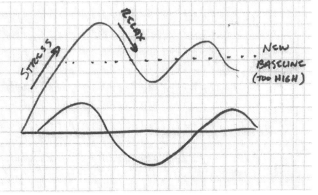

Diagram 1.2

Tim's body actually maladapts to the amount of chronic stress he feels in his environment. He's always expecting danger, so his body follows suit. His baseline becomes elevated (Diagram 1.2), and he starts to become constantly agitated or irritated. He can't focus on a task because his mind is always looking for the next threat. His physiology mirrors this as his sympathetic nervous system is continually activated.

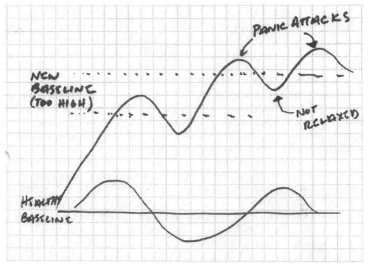

Diagram 1.3

With that constant activation, he can't relax at the poker table. He can't even pause and appreciate that his Vegas trip is supposed to energize him. Instead, he's so fired up that the smallest danger (in this case, the possibility of losing, even just a few dollars) becomes overblown. He starts to pant, and he feels lightheaded. A panic attack is just the next step in his over-activated sympathetic nervous system (Diagram 1.3)

The focus of this book is on the parasympathetic system, which is the counterpart to Tim's overactive sympathetic system. In the latter state, Tim has difficulty slowing down. With his baseline so high, Tim has to spend time – through habits, rituals, techniques, etc. – in lowering it. It's something doable, and it's the focus of this book.

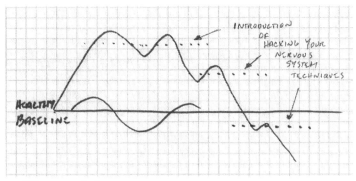

Diagram 1.4

With this book, I aim to provide you with multiple breathing, body position, and psychological (mind) techniques that can help you slow down. Hopefully, we can get your stress wave to more like a natural balance like Diagram 1.1:

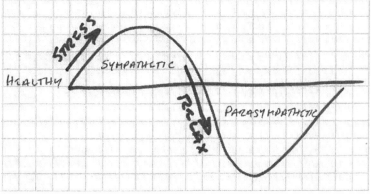

Diagram 1.1

So let's see what would happen if Tim's situation played out a little differently. Let's imagine him equipped with some of the techniques in this book. Let's see how he would approach the stressed-out poker table with the knowledge of working on his breath, eating the right foods, cultivating the correct body posture, and managing his mental state and emotions. He would have the tools to modulate his ANS.

It would go something like this:

Tim sees a poker table. He's excited at the possibility of winning money, but he also recognizes that he could lose easily. It's risky, and he feels his heart beating, faster and faster. His palms are starting to sweat, but instead of sitting down and trying to order a drink, Tim pauses and closes his eyes. He remembers his body is primitively scanning for threats and is in a heightened mode. He uses the same covert techniques used by hostage negotiators which you'll learn in Chapter 2. While doing this, he becomes aware of his shallow breathing. As his heart rate starts to slow down, he straightens his back and assumes a power pose (that you'll soon learn). He feels a little more confident knowing that his daily exercises (including this stance) can influence his hormones and, consequently, his physiology. As he opens his eyes, he feels lighter.

He smiles and walks toward the poker table and assumes a confident position as he stretches his arms out. The other onlookers also notice his calm demeanor and are drawn to him. Tim understands that he also has to be wary of what goes into his body, both physical and psychological. He notes that he should probably abstain or try to avoid sugary drinks. He also wants not to feel as sluggish with an alcoholic drink, so he opts for a water. Even with the game starting, Tim remembers that this is just a game. He feels pangs of anxiety and stress – but he was expecting them. His mind is starting to echo his body, and his body is also telling his mind (through his ANS), that he's okay.

This practice of hacking his nervous system may help him win more rounds of poker and also enjoy more of life. Learning to click out of turbo mode will allow him to fully enjoy the profits.

We should not live in a constant state of anxiety or heightened awareness. We deserve a body and a mind that can not only handle modern stressors, but also thrive in any environment. I wish to impart to you various techniques that I know will be invaluable in your toolkit. What follows is a general overview of the book – along the way you'll be learning some of my favorite hacks.

Chapter 2 will be an overview of breathing techniques. For example, I'll share with you a technique used by snipers and hostage negotiators to slow down your racing thoughts and focus on the task at hand. I've taught the techniques to stressed parents, executives, and teens with ADHD

Chapter 3 will be an overview of body posture and how it affects your mood and cognition. You'll learn some techniques that work well below public speeches or when you want to gain power.

Chapter 4 will be on the mind. We'll discuss the importance of mindfulness and how stress affects the various parts of the brain. Plus, we'll talk about the evolution of both your mind and brain.

Each of the next few chapters will also have an associated exercise at the end. It will be a summary of what techniques we have uncovered in our time together. I hope that it will be a quick of way of getting you from theory to action. But they require practice and diligence! My goal is for you to implement these tools on a day-to-day basis.

Journal Exercises

You should look at journaling as logging your own story. This is an excellent way for immediate feedback as it helps to clarify mental blocks. You might uncover ideas or patterns in various thoughts that you should commit to writing. It's also an excellent way for your mind to be focused and primed.

Here are some thoughts:

When was the last time you felt very stressed out? Write down three thoughts or feelings associated with that moment.

What does stress mean to you? How do you usually deal with it?

Summary

- The body's nervous system is an intricate web of anatomical structures and neurochemical messengers that help with our perceptions of the world.

- Modern stressors have affected our physiology, and we need tools to help modulate our autonomic nervous system.
- Sympathetic system: Fight or flight (gas pedal, on/go mode).
- Parasympathetic system: Rest and digest (brake pedal, of/slow mode).
- Stress will always be there, but we can generate habits, rituals, and techniques to help reduce the extreme variations between the sympathetic and parasympathetic systems.

Chapter 2: Breath

Breath is the rhythm of life.
— Hippocratic aphorism

When the National Academics Defense Centers of Excellence for Psychological Health and Traumatic Brain Injury conducted a study named "Mind-body Techniques for Regulating the Autonomic Nervous System (ANS)," breathing was the first recommended method. Why? How you breathe has a profound impact on your mind and body.

Think back to Tim's casino experience. In Tim's case, when he was stressed out, he was breathing incorrectly. Tim's hyperactive sympathetic nervous system saw the threat at the poker table. The body went into a reactive mode and began either over-breathing (usually through the mouth) or under-breathing (to be fully silent). So the solution is simple, right? Just breath smoother, deeper, and slower. Maybe just use your lungs to the fullest capacity?

Unfortunately, no. Breathing is so much more than that.

In order to really understand how our ANS and breathing go hand in hand, we need to briefly (don't worry, it won't be painful!) explore how our own biochemistry with oxygen affects the former. To make it more interesting, let's talk about sex!

Wait...What? Yes, that's right: we can use intercourse as a segue into the unique relationship between breath and the parasympathetic nervous system.

––––––––––––––––

In our previous discussion of the ANS and the vagus nerve, I included a chart that highlighted the differences between the two systems. In the "Sexual/Reproductive" aspect, the parasympathetic system is known for prolonging the sexual and orgasm experience. In the sympathetic system, intercourse isn't vital to the immediate survival needs of the organism. So there's vaginal dryness and either less potency or rapid ejaculation.

In order to get into this more sensual and parasympathetic state, we need exercises to stimulate the vagus nerve. The good news is we can use breathing to start this process.

When you breathe deeply and hold your breath, it increases your intra-abdominal pressure. This is the pressure within your abdominal cavity. There are certain receptors called "baroreceptors" that sense this change. With increased pressure levels, baroreceptors send signals to the vagus nerve. It gets activated and sends signals of relaxation throughout your body.

In fact, with continual practice, these baroreceptors, or stretch receptors, get better over time. Your ANS gets more sensitive to these techniques, and your parasympathetic system can get activated more efficiently (Jereth et al., 2006).

So what does that mean for your sex life?

In order for you to have a long session of sex, you need to inhale through the nose to stimulate the vagus nerve. If you want even more calming energy, as you exhale, make any sound your body feels like making — a grunt, a groan, a moan. The more excited you get, the louder the sound.

You can see then that the breath has such an integral part of your own stress and ANS. So deep, smooth breaths can really make the difference in your own well-being and activate your ANS for your own benefit — and under your own terms. But we should also explore the opposite: short, shallow breathing....

Are You Fear Breathing?

Let's take a moment and observe how you're breathing. Are you using the full lungs by breathing into the belly? Or is it a shallow breath that is only filling the top of the lungs? Are you using your mouth or your nose? Is the breathing rhythmic or stuttered? The differences in breathing style — how you're breathing — can have a huge impact on your health and wellbeing.

At its worst, "fear breathing" is unconsciously holding our breath. Recall the last time you were seriously scared. Maybe you thought you heard someone in the house, someone sneak up on you, or you thought you'd lost a wallet or valuable item. Chances are you held your breath.

Fear breath is unhealthy for us because it encourages the fight-flight branch of the nervous system.

In *The Breath Connection*, professor Robert Fried (1990) argues about the sympathetic nervous system and holding our breath. He states that a "fear reaction invariably involves breath holding; the release of hormones into the blood causing reduced blood flow to the extremities, increased heart rate and blood pressure, automatic muscular blood flow adjustments, and involuntary changes in digestive and other internal organs (p. 39)."

It's the opposite of the slower breathing we talked about earlier.

When we experience fear, consciously or subconsciously, we hold or reduce our breathing rate. Breath holding brings the body out of the parasympathetic mode and more into the sympathetic state. This movement of blood toward the muscles is great if you need to run from a lion or find yourself fighting an attacker. However, fear breath is bad for regular life. It's not good for the boardroom, and it's bad for the bedroom. Let's talk about why.

Fear breath may discourage weight loss.

Researchers at University of New South Wales found that fat primarily exits the body through the breath. Fat gets broken down into carbon, which is bound to a pair of oxygen molecules and exhaled. According to the study, if you examine "10 kilograms of fat as they are 'lost', 8.4 of those kilograms are exhaled as carbon dioxide through the lungs. The remaining 1.6 kilograms becomes water, which may be excreted in urine, feces, sweat, breath, tears and other bodily fluids" (Meerman, 2014).

Maybe our failure to breathe fully could be a contributing factor to the US obesity epidemic.

Fear breath may cause DNA dreadlocks.

Picture DNA, the strands of chromosomes that are our bodies' blueprints, as strands of hair. On the end of each strand is an end cap that prevents split ends. This is called a telomere. Recent science has shown that, when lung function is reduced and when we have more shallow breaths, it has the effect of shortening these telomeres (Albrecht et al., 2014). When these telomeres shorten, we age faster at a cellular level because the split ends cause damage and unhealthy binding of DNA strands. Those damaged DNA strands get copied, resulting in more damaged, weathered cells.

Maybe breathing the right way also modulates the way we age.

Fear breath may be bad for sex and reproduction.

That's right. When we are in fight-flight, all blood flow moves toward survival functions and away from non-critical functions — including reproduction. There is reduced blood flow to the non-critical body parts, including the sexual organs. The body is in a fear reactive state and less likely to have the full reproductive functions.

Maybe holding our breath is sabotaging our sex life.

Fear breath may encourage bad breath.

Here's the theory: When we don't breathe deeply, we don't expel much carbon dioxide. Carbon dioxide is acidic. So our acid/alkaline balance slides toward acidity. Typically, harmful bacteria, like those that cause bad breath, grow in more acidic environments. Full deep breaths will expel more of the acidity through exhales, promoting an alkalinity in the body that doesn't support negative bacteria growth (Toletino et al., 2011). The absence of positive bacteria contributes to bad breath. Additionally, when we mouth breathe, we're more likely to dry the mouth, which is intended to remain moist to allow the good bacteria to flourish.

_____

We've examined ways that shallow breathing — aka "fear breathing," which is a natural reaction of the body to fight-flight or stressful situations — is bad for health.

Performance experts have known for some time that breathing affects our mental and physical performance.

That's why people preparing to be in critical positions (hostage negotiators, professional athletes, and moms giving birth) are taught how to be cognizant of their breathing and to practice techniques. By retraining their breathing, they can enhance performance, focus on the tasks at hand, and relax amid high stress.

In the next section, I'll share with you some of these same exercises so that you can combat fear breath in your day-to-day life.

Caution

A note of caution: Irregular breathing may be a sign of a medical condition, so before beginning this or any other exercise program, you should consult with a doctor to see if there's any underlying condition that needs to be addressed.

With any of these exercises, it's also important to adopt this mindset: *Slow is smooth and smooth is fast.* It's a saying attributed to the Navy SEALs and the way they take on habits and learning.

We should learn these skills slowly, each of us observing our own body's reactions. We shouldn't be harsh on ourselves if we don't accomplish them at the first try. We want consistency. My goal is for you to learn these skills and get better over time. Then you can incorporate this into your daily practice.

RISE Method

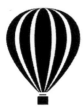

So what's the antidote to FEAR Breath? Let's RISE above fear with the RISE method.

A relaxing, healthy breath consists of 4 parts:

Relax   the abdomen and pelvic region
Inhale   deeply through the nose
Sound   observe the sound and sensation in the body
Exhale through the nose

Try that now.

Repeat this type of breathing for a few minutes.

Relax. When we get stressed, we tense up the belly and the pelvic region. The first part of this breathing is to relax the belly and let the stomach out so that the lungs can expand fully. When we relax and breathe fully into the abdominal cavity, then we allow the vagus nerve to get stimulated. Remember those baroreceptors feeling the change in abdominal pressure? They send signals to the vagus nerve to put the body into the parasympathetic mode.

Inhale. The second part is to inhale deeply through the nose. Inhaling through the nose allows the body to filter and humidify the air to a more comfortable level for the lungs. In fact, research has shown that breathing through the nose stimulates parasympathetic function (Telles et al., 1993).

Sound and Sensation. The third part is to either observe the sounds of your breath or your environment. Notice the sensations in the body.

During times of stress, we lose our present-moment thinking.

We dabble either in anxiety and thinking about the future — or we lament and wallow about the past.

But when we observe the sounds of the breath, we are brought back to the present moment. Observe the coolness of the breath in the nose. Maybe the warmth of the breath in the lungs. Feel the pelvic region, the stomach.

We can also use this time to make a sound. Making a sound is also called "resistance breathing." It helps us to both stimulate more parasympathetic function and discharge some of the stress that is in the body.

When we're sick, for example, we moan, and that moaning feels good to do. Another example is the Om. Om-ing has a very powerful influence on the brain. A cat purrs, and that's a good sign that it's going to a parasympathetic or calming place. For thousands of years, yogis and other cultures have chanted and used music as a way to calibrate the responses of the body (Vickhoff, 2013). It's said that if you're approaching vasovagal syncope (or about to faint), and you chant the Ave Maria or a yogic chant, you're more likely not to faint (Bernadi 2001). Breathing truly is the rhythm of life as Hippocrates said.

Resistance breathing can be performed simply with some humming sounds when we exhale. It's hard to stay angry or stressed while humming.

Exhale. The fourth part is to exhale, either through the nose or through the mouth, if you want to be more mindful. Exhale fully and deeply — without force or pressure.

Exhale in such a way that it doesn't build up in the mouth.

When we breathe deeply into the belly (aka diaphragmatic) and take time for these conscious breaths, science suggests that it decreases cortisol and increases the antioxidants in the body (Martarelli et al., 2011). This is especially helpful for faster recovery during intense workouts.

During any tense or stressful moment, taking the time to be conscious of the breath will help defuse the stress.

Parachute Breath

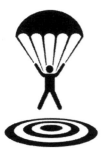

When the mind is racing out of control, we're probably in a fight-flight mode. We're probably feeling stressed and maybe feeling either defensive or reactive. That means that we're in more of a sympathetic mode of our nervous system. Remember that the exhale is a parasympathetic movement. It calms the body. Each inhale energizes the body and gives us life, and it's borne of slight fear. Each exhale relaxes the body and brings us into a calmer place.

When you're feeling like the mind is racing out of control, and you need to slow things down:

1. Take a deep breath in through the nose.

2. Hold it briefly. Then inhale a bit more.

3. Pause and very slowly exhale through the mouth.

4. Repeat up to three to four times.

This is the same reason it's hard to be angry and anxious while you're whistling or humming. The whistling action and the humming action slows the breath down. The longer it slows the exhale down, and the longer you can slow the exhale down, the more relaxed you'll be. This is one of those techniques that needs practice, so try it a few times, perhaps before meditation. Then you'll be able to use it when stress hits you. The reason I call it "parachute breath" is that the parachute slows the person down by slowing the flow of air through it. You can think of the exhale as being a very ... slowing of the mind.

The Gravity Breath

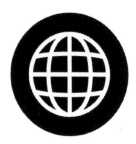

Before I explain this powerful technique, let me first explain an interesting finding: According to an article in the *Journal of Experimental Biology,* "in diving mammals and heavy exercisers, the spleen serves as an oxygen reservoir, storing highly viscous 'thick blood', rich in red blood cells, during periods of rest, and injecting these stored red blood cells into the general circulation when oxygen levels are stressed and increased transport is required" (Milton, 2004). So it may be that the spleen acts as an oxygen backpack that we can use before stressful times.

How to do the Gravity Breath

1. Full inhale through nose.
2. Exhale through the mouth. Just a letting go of breath. Not necessary to fully exhale.
3. Repeat for 30-40 deep breaths.
4. Exhale out and HOLD after this last exhale out for as long as possible.
5. Deep inhale and hold for 10 seconds.

6. Exhale and resume normal breathing.

When?
I do this in the morning, before or after something stressful like a presentation or negotiation. That way I am full of oxygen and can perform better.

  This technique is adapted from one of my teachers, Wim Hof.

Box Breathing

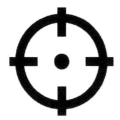

Let's say you're in a long, stressful meeting. You want a method to steady the mind and focus your attention. We can borrow a technique used by some special forces members or snipers.

Box breathing is used to calm the nervous system. Traditionally, it's a count of 4 for all sides of the box. But I've found that extending the exhale counts helps to calm the body.

1. Inhale for a count of 4.
2. Hold for a count of 4.
3. Exhale for a count of 6.
4. Hold for a count of 2.

What to do when exercising?

As an aside, I would suggest breathing through the nose while you're training. When you're in a competition and you need to turn up the juice a little bit, for a short burst, you can switch to mouth breathing. But overall, you want to train to breathe through the nose. If you find that you're not able to breathe hard enough, then you need to slow down the exercise. When you're in a period where you need to relax, then you want to breathe through the nose, deep full breaths. This includes when you're in the boardroom, bedroom, and everywhere in between.

Conclusion & Take Ten

Next time you're happy, take note of your breathing.

Notice how full and expanded your breath is. How it fills the lungs, deeply.

Notice when you look at a baby: the belly expands and contracts. This happens as the lungs grow in size with each breath, pushing the stomach out. Take a moment and see, feel the front of the lungs, and then imagine breathing into the back of the lungs and letting the stomach hang out.

It's helpful to take ten minutes to breathe and relax, taking full deep breaths in through the nose, into the belly, and exhaling with a sound. Any sound will do. Take ten minutes before leaving for the day, ten minutes before or after eating to put the body into a relaxed state, which will boost digestion. Then take ten minutes when you come home from work or before sex when you need to relax. Ten minutes of deep, full breaths.

Let's go back to the story of our poker player, Tim. What would he have done differently? Rather than panicking at the stress and uncertainty of the game, he would slow down. He would take a deep breath. He would be transported to the present moment as his breath becomes an anchor. He would have understanding that hyperventilating with shallow breaths is only revving up his sympathetic system. Maybe he would excuse himself and find somewhere quiet to breathe. Or during the game, he would consciously choose to breathe deeply. He would appreciate that the bigger breaths he is taking are activating receptors that signal his parasympathetic system. Slowly, the fear would give way to relaxation.

Summary

- Deep breathing activates the parasympathetic system through stretching of the baroreceptors.
- Fear breathing is an extension of the sympathetic system and has a variety of negative side effects.
- Learning how to breathe is a skill that can be developed and improved over time.

When in doubt, don't fret.
Just breathe.
Deep out.
Deep in.

"Feelings come and go like clouds in a windy sky. Conscious breathing is my anchor."
— **Thich Nhat Hanh, Stepping into Freedom: Rules of Monastic Practice for Novices**

Chapter 3: Body

You should pray for a healthy mind in a healthy body.
Ask for a stout heart that has no fear of death, and deems length of days the least of Nature's gifts
that can endure any kind of toil,
— Roman poet Juvenal

Tim's at the poker table with his hands clenched. His eyes squint as he tries to tell himself to "focus." He feels warm and thinks that the other people around him can see his flushed face. He's hunched over. His head is low and keeps to himself. All he can just do is play the game. But he's fidgeting around, and he feels thirsty. His stomach starts to growl, and his lower back starts to ache. He can't stop tapping his foot. It's his nerves. It has to be. He is scared. He's shaken — he almost lost the last hand. He can feel the pulse in his legs and in his thighs.

_____

We know Tim because we see people like him everywhere. We recognize their physical movements: posture, gait, voice intonation, facial expressions, personal space. All of these are samples of their internal state. These are cues to what they're feeling inside. Sometimes stress will also freeze a person's affect.

We call this body language, or a style of nonverbal communication that stresses physical behavior. We look at other people to decode their emotions. Some studies show that up to 93% — 93%!!! — of all communication is nonverbal (Mehrabian, 1967). We pay attention to the way people sit, the tone of their voice, the symmetry of their smile — maybe even their posture when they hear bad news.

Whenever we are in a stressful situation, our bodies also talk. The body adapts to the thoughts and ideas that are racing through your head whenever you see a looming figure in the background. Or maybe that car crash you just avoided. Fear and the ANS can shape your physique.

Our minds can sculpt the way we hold our bodies.

Fear Body

When we are in fear our body contracts.

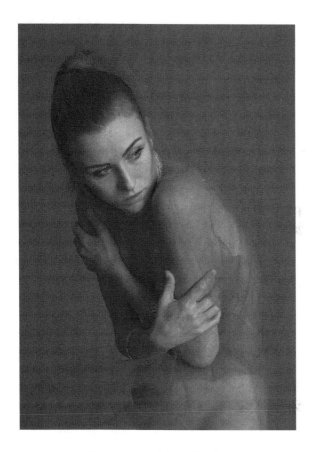

Here are a few signs of fear body:
- Not taking up space
- Chest is going inward
- Neck hangs forward
- Touching your neck
- Tight lower back and pelvis
- Looking down and away
- Not breathing fully into the belly

Why does the body act this way?

Because fear causes the ANS to put the body into a protective or defensive position. The ANS is intertwined with muscle fibers throughout the body. Some fibers control breathing. Others control posture. And some even control muscle strength and the way we talk.

We contract to provide tension to attack, run away, or lessen the surface area that can be struck. This action happens unconsciously.

Here's a simple model* of how this works:

Stressor -> Fear -> Amygdala ->Hypothalamus -> Sympathetic nervous system -> Acute response

* The neuroanatomy of fear is much more comprehensive. It includes other regions of the brain and how our memories can also tinge our experiences. For the sake of our discussion, it's best we just choose a more streamlined process.

Let's break down each component.

Stressor: A stressor is whatever stimuli that causes you to be afraid. It can be a shadowy figure following you late at night. Or a dreaded meeting with your regional manager about your job. A vibration of the cell phone. A text from a family member. Or even that exam looming in the horizon. It doesn't have to be physical. It doesn't even have to be real. In fact, the brain sometimes even comprehends fake fears as much as real ones.

The amygdala: This is an almond-shaped area of the brain that deals with emotional processing. You see something scary, and this structure sends out distress signals.

The hypothalamus: We can think of this part of the brain as a command station. It relays the messages from the amygdala that have been tinged with emotions and even past memories. It sends these messages to the sympathetic arm of the ANS.

Sympathetic: This is the "fight/flight" system of the ANS we have already been talking about. It's a collection of nerves and hormones that sends signals to put the body into a more active role. Remember the diagram 1.2 in chapter 1? This is the typical response: heart racing, flushing, sweating, blood pumping through your veins, and testosterone and other hormones surging through your body.

Acute response: This is just the sympathetic response that you have. It can be the choice to run away or to fight back — or to sweat profusely or just freeze.

To account for this, here's what I think happens:

Stressor -> Fear -> Amygdala -> Hypothalamus ->
Sympathetic nervous system -> Chronic response ->
   Fear body

In Amy Cuddy's seminal Ted Talk, "Your Body Language Shapes Who You Are," we were introduced to a model of how our physical state (posture, body position, etc.) can influence our emotional state. Traditionally, the belief is that the mind affects the body's functions. When we feel shame, fear, anger, or guilt, it can manifest in the body. Think about how psychological fatigue can tense up our shoulders. Most people think that just focusing on the mind (see the next chapter) will ameliorate stress and the way it affects the body — but this is only part of the puzzle.

Cuddy's research shows that, when we move the body in certain postures, it can affect the ANS. She proposed a certain set of postures and movements called "power poses" that modulates our neurohormonal systems, which in turns affects our emotional state.

In other words, how we move our bodies and how we orient ourselves in space can affect how we feel about stress.

Expanding the body sends signals to the nervous system. It tells the body to reduce cortisol levels and increase testosterone. It helps to explain why these individuals in Cuddy's experiment felt less stressed (lower cortisol) and were more confident and more likely to take risks (testosterone).

A formula for power can be defined as:

> *High testosterone + low cortisol = High power*
>
> *Low testosterone + high cortisol = Low power*

But how does this fit within the fear body? Well, I think Amy Cuddy's ideas on this expanded cognition can lead the way to how we approach chronic stress in the body. We can reprogram the body by consciously changing our posture and the way we take up space in the world, and presumably, we can get the body out of this fear contortion.

Here's another way of looking at it.

Stressor -> Fear -> Amygdala -> Hypothalamus -> Sympathetic nervous system -> Chronic response -> Lower status poses -> Fear body -> Power poses -> Positive neurohormonal feedback-> Heathier emotional state

Take up space unapologetically.
Expand your presence.

Thus, by being aware you are in your "fear body" and taking the steps to fix your posture and body position by employing Cuddy's power poses and other techniques (which will come next), you can realign your neurohormonal system and, thus, get into a better mood.

Power Poses

Here is a list of some power poses you can do before or during stressful moments. Sometimes, all you need is just two minutes. Try to do these in front of a mirror. Maybe you can imagine your favorite actor or actress doing this beside you. However you do it, you want to make this a habit. Over time, your body will start to unconsciously do these postures and poses. Even during times of stress, you'll start to retrain yourself to become more powerful and have a stronger presence.

1. Superman or Wonder Woman Pose

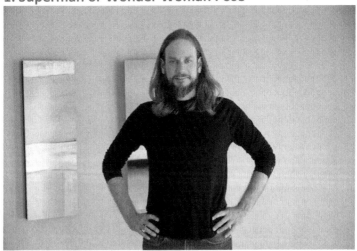

- Stand up straight puffing your chest slightly out.
- Put your hands or fists to your side.
- Breathe in.
- Breathe out.

- Spend 2 minutes in this pose.

This is a good one to do before an anxiety provoking experience like a public talk.

2. Stake Out the Table

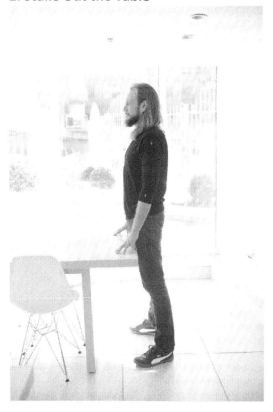

- Make sure both hands are open, loose.
- Relax your shoulders.
- Plant both feet on the ground, shoulder width apart.

- Leading with your waist, lean into the side of a table.
- Put both your hands on the table to hold you.
- Look straight ahead and hold the pose for 2 minutes.

3. Leaning in During Conversations

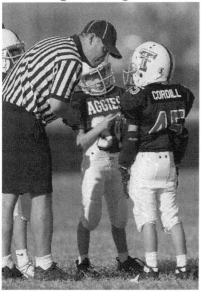

This is a good one to do when you're trying to make a point or if you feel like you are losing ground in a conversation.

- Lean in whenever you're talking to someone. (Not in a creepy or intrusive way).
- Or lean in and try to hear the person who is talking in a group conversation.

4. Victory Pose

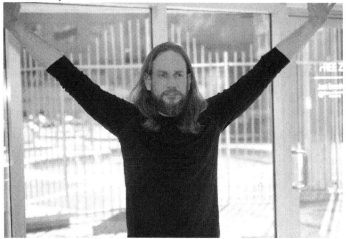

- Put your hands up in the air (like the people in an awards ceremony).
- Become aware of your full, deep breaths.
- Close your eyes and think of the last time you've won something — or some great celebration.
- Hold your hands up for 30 seconds or more.

5. Taking Up Your Chair Space

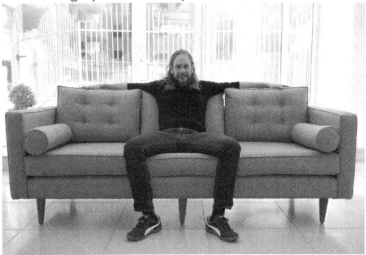

This is one of my favorites. And it's something I like to do before stressful meetings. Or doctor's appointments. Or job interviews.

- Find an open area to sit, preferably somewhere with two or three chairs.
- Sit in the middle chair.
- Move your butt and back up against the back of the chair.
- Put your hands and arms on adjacent chairs.
- Lean your head back.
- Cross your legs in a 90-degree angle.
- Relax, breathe in, breathe out.

Chronic Fear Body & Lower Back Pain

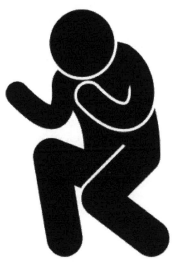

The body's response to fear is automatic and unconscious. When the threat is detected, the body goes deeper into fight/flight automatically. The major muscles to fight or flight are in the pelvic region. They serve to lower our center of gravity, crouch down to protect the gut, or get the body ready to run. The most important of these muscle is the "fight/flight" muscle – the psoas.

As I said earlier, we live in a culture of constant stress and anxiety. Through our connected world, we are constantly being bombarded with images, news, ideas, and information that can paralyze us. Our access to knowledge has made us that much more aware to potential danger in our surroundings. This ongoing exposure chronically triggers the impulse to fight or flight. Turbo mode gets us ready to run from a saber tooth tigers. When stress and fear is chronic, we are stuck in turbo or a high state of alert. Tension stays present in the body in order to react at a moments notice to the looming threat.

Unfortunately, a lot of that tension is based in the pelvis. When stress hits, you literally become a tight ass. And with chronic stress, we may stay that way.

Let's explore the psoas which is the core of the fight/flight response and the cause of a lot of back pain.

The Psoas

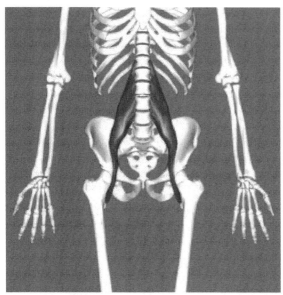

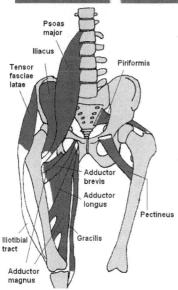

Psoas major

Iliacus

Tensor fasciae latae

Piriformis

Adductor brevis

Adductor longus

Pectineus

Iliotibial tract

Gracilis

Adductor magnus

The psoas is a fascinating muscle located deep within the pelvic region. It connects the femur, or upper leg, to the lumbar region of the spine. That's your lower back. The lower back has vertebrae, bones, and disks, which are like jelly-filled bubbles. In fact, the lumbar region is an area that tends to have a lot of lower back surgeries. When we feel stress, the psoas tightens and becomes tense. This tension can be released improperly and can lead to structural issues down the road. This can include damaging those fragile, jelly-filled disks.

Think about the last time you missed a step. Your body automatically goes into a position of contracting the abdomen and heads toward the thighs to roll you into a ball to protect the head and the belly. One of the first muscles that fires, or contracts, is the psoas, and it pulls the rest of the body into this protective position. This affects the muscles in the back and even the diaphragm and neck. When the diaphragm contracts this way, it results in shallower breathing. And as we discussed in chapter two, these shallower breaths increase stress.

So when you tighten the body and the psoas, so too does the mechanics of your breathing change. As a result, we don't activate our parasympathetic system through our vagus nerve. Rather, we are continually activating our sympathetic system, which only worsens our stress and mood, and tightens our lower back and pelvic region.

Furthermore, the psoas is not easily manipulated by a massage therapist or other muscular maneuvers as it's deep within the pelvic region and is very close to the sexual organs. It's not easy to unwind. When there is harm done, such as a psoas tear or similar, individuals are bedridden (to help allow the muscle to heal), and they tend to feel anxiety, fear or anger, and low back pain. Stress can't be released properly from these damaged structures. I believe that these symptoms are related to holding all these feelings, manifesting in dread and distress.

Thus, the "fear body" is the physical manifestation of long-standing fear/stress. In order to really understand why the body acts this way (fetal position, poor posture, small space), we have to consider our core and, particularly, the psoas. In *Shake It Off*, Robert Scaer eloquently captures this idea:

In any threatening experience, the neck muscles will pull the neck forward, the shoulder muscles will raise the shoulders and draw them inward, and the hip girdle muscles will flex the hip toward the abdomen and curve the spine, pulling the pelvis up toward the abdomen. All of these movements are hard-wired in the brains of all creatures for the purpose of drawing the body inward to protect the front of the neck, the chest and abdomen. This is known as the fetal response. It is the safest position of the human body and it replicates the position of the fetus (p. IX).

But we shouldn't lament at our physiology. Instead, we should embrace the idea that we too can sculpt our own bodies. In the same way that stress can modulate our posture and the way we hold ourselves in the world, we too can do the same. We can play an active role in how we hold ourselves, and we can see that paying attention to our physical state can affect our mood. We can develop habits and techniques to not only release the psoas, but make our bodies more limber, loose and able to handle uncertainty.

The most powerful method of psoas release I can find will be covered in a follow-on video in the Hacking Your Nervous System series: the TRMR.

For now, let's take a look at another one of my favorites: Constructive Rest Position.

Constructive Rest Position

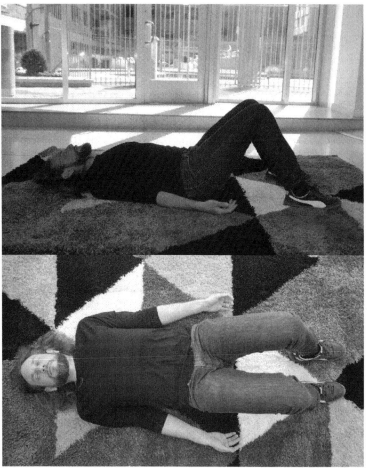

The constructive rest position is a gravitational release of the abdominal muscles. It primarily relaxes the psoas and other major core muscles that are usually more tense due to chronic stress.

- Lay on your back on the floor.
- Put your heels hip width apart.

- Keep your feet flat on the floor.
- Allow your arms to rest on the floor.
- Feel the sensations of your body, back, and core muscles.
- Do nothing and relax.

Yup, that's right.

We want to just relax and stay in this position. You might feel some discomfort. It might feel awkward. But that's the years of stress and other bad programming that's affected these regions of the body. Try to push through the discomfort. Just a little bit.

Just start off for about 5 minutes a day. Maybe in the morning. Maybe at night. But you want to keep doing this and build up your resistance.

Here is a good schedule you can follow. As you get stronger and your body gets used to this position, it will get easier. The sensations will get better, and you will get into a relaxed state much faster.

Week 1: 5 minutes
Week 2: 10 minutes
Week 3: 15 minutes
Week 4: 20 minutes
Week 5: 25 minutes
Week 6: 30 minutes

———————

Other Techniques

Here's a list of other small techniques that I like to show clients to help loosen up the body.

Massage the Head

Another way to clear the head of toxins is to massage the top sides of the head using your fingernails to lightly scratch or stimulate on the skin. On the neck, continue down onto the neck, back of the neck, the front of the neck, massaging with your fingertips, the soft side of your fingertips, brushing downward as you're doing that. That helps open up the lymphatic system of the head, and by moving the skin around, you help move the craniosacral fluid of the body. Movement of these fluids may allow the body to properly hydrate and flush toxins.

Neck Rolls

The other thing that's helpful is to do slow neck rolls, three to four neck rolls in each direction, and stretch out the neck. That helps release any stiffness in this important connection point between the brain and the body.

Relax the Eyes and Eyebrows

The eyes and eyebrows are another source of tension in the body and face. When somebody is angry or upset, the eyebrows get closer together, and there's that wrinkle that appears. According to Ayurveda, an Indian mind-body health system, this may be a sign that somebody is angry, upset, or in a sympathetic mode or stressed-out mode. What we can do is closing our eyes and relaxing a point between eyebrows which will help relax the muscles around. Just feel the stress and tension dissolving around the eyes now that they are closed.

Release the Jaw and Relax the Tongue

Another great method that works is to open and relax the jaw, and move the jaw from side to side. There may be some clicking noises or discomfort, so spend a few moments relaxing the jaw, then relaxing the inside of the face, and noticing any tension that exists in the tongue region. Relaxing the tongue and allowing some space between the tongue and the roof of the mouth is one of the stealth techniques that can be used in meetings. When you're stressed, just relax and wobble the tongue around in the center in the mouth. According to Chinese medicine, the tongue is connected to every part of the body, and as we relax the tongue, the rest of the body will relax.

Drop the Shoulders

Make a point to consciously drop the shoulders and chest when you're stressed. The fear response is for the shoulders to come upward to protect the neck and bring us forward. But with practice, if you drop the shoulders down lightly, you feel more relaxed. You don't hold the tension in this part of the body. Your upper body feels more loose.

Practice. Practice. Practice.
With all of these things, it's like brushing your teeth. Every day you have to do it. You'll notice that you'll want to brush your teeth once for the rest of your life. You'll want to relax your tongue once for the rest of your life. That doesn't happen. These are all practices to return to, and you're not going to permanently relax the tongue, relax the eyebrows, or relax the lower back. So practice!

Conclusion

At the end of the day, fear and stress don't just exist in the mind. They can spill into the body and cause it to become rigid and stiff. Poor posture and chronic stressors can sculpt the way we hold our bodies. This causes negative feedback loops that affect our ANS and our mood.

In order to fix this, we need to focus on the body. We need to get out of the fear body state. We need to develop the habit or ritual of these power poses. These tools instruct the mind through the body that we are powerful. We need our physicality to signal the mind that we aren't small and that we are confident.

Let's imagine Tim with some of these techniques down. Instead of sitting down hunched over the table, you would see him confidently sit down. His chest is puffed, and he's leaning in as he's telling the dealer he is going to join the game. He smiles at the beautiful woman at the side of the table, and he relaxes his back. His arms wrap over two extra chairs as he sits crossed-legs. His body language shows that he's open and ready to accept whatever happens. These movements signal to his body that's he's ready. Tim's stress melts away as he feels a pang of confidence (or testosterone) slowly building up. The game begins, and Tim announces, rather than meekly nodding, what he wants to do next.

The ANS is not only affected by our thinking, but also by our actions and behaviors. And thus, by doing these power poses or other techniques, we can shape our perception of ourselves and the mind will follow.

Summary

- Stress can be stored in the muscles and especially in the abdominal, pelvic, and psoas areas.
- You can perform a variety of postures and poses that help to modulate a variety of neurohormonal responses.
- You can actually practice these power poses to help out with stress and relaxation.

Chapter 4: Mind

Not everyone can see the extent of Tim's stress. Over the years, he has become a master of the poker face – concealing the chaos and tension inside his body and mind. But, Tim is stressed out and his mind is racing out of control. His breathing is irregular. His back is tense. He's constantly irritated by the way the poker game is going. The smallest distraction, a small conversation, even a smile, takes him out of the zone. He can't concentrate, and he feels restless. His body is aching from the restrained stress that has been building up in his abdominal and lower back region. Even more so, his short and shallow breaths are still priming his sympathetic system.

People may be reading Tim's tense body language, but no one knows what's really going on in his mind. Even Tim is unaware of how narrow-minded and fear-based his mind has become. In the same way that our bodies can shape our minds, even the way we perceive stress and anxiety can actually color our perception of the world and sculpt the way our minds work. The irony is that he *knows* he's stressed out. But the brief moments of awareness are washed away by a constant barrage of negative thoughts and emotions ("What if I lose this money?" "Why am I so stressed out?" "Did I forget something?" "Why didn't they laugh at my joke?" "Should I fold or just try to push my hand?" "Wait...What was I thinking again?").

Tim doesn't know that he's so stressed out. He has lost self-awareness. Let me say that again: Tim's stress has affected his overall moment-to-moment awareness. It's compromised, and he won't perform well. He can't focus on his thoughts. Nor can he evaluate them. He knows that the stress is affecting his cognition. But he can't even see that it has narrowed his perception of the world. He doesn't know that he is thinking in a fear and scarcity mindset whereby everything (even a small stimulus like a misplaced poker hand) immediately jolts his sympathetic system.

He knows that he has to do something. But the stress and anxiety have overwhelmed him.

The previous chapters (Breathing and Body) focused on the external manifestations of the ANS. We've discussed how chronic stress states affect breathing patterns and body postures. This constant anxiety has as real of an effect on our physiology as on our breathing (via baroreceptors for example) and even on our posture (via the neurohormonal feedback by body poses).

But what about the mind? What happens with chronic stress and anxiety and the way it affects the mind and its interaction with the sympathetic and parasympathetic systems? As I explained earlier, this chapter will focus on the idea of the fear mindset. In the same vein that the earlier chapters have woven a story of fear-based breathing and body postures, so too will this chapter explore how fear contorts the mind.

In order to understand how the mind reacts to fear, we have to take a few steps back. We have to go back to the beginning, before our ANS was born, before a lot of the neural networks that surge through our body were established. We have to start this conversation when the brain was first formed.

So let's talk delve into some evolutionary neurobiology. Don't worry! We won't be slogging through details.

We can imagine the development of the brain by the formation of three layers. This is called the "triune" brain theory. Each layer has a specific name and a specific function. As evolution has formed the brain's neural networks, so too has it built up the various layers of the brain.

We will explore each layer and see how it fits within an evolutionary timeline and framework. And more importantly, it will literally (no pun intended!) lay the foundation as to why our minds are warped by fear.

The 3 Layers of the Triune Brain

The first layer is the reptilian brain. It's the oldest of the three layers. It is responsible for primitive behavioral patterns necessary for survival of self and species (Gould, 2003). This basic layer is involved with the 4 F's : Feeding, fighting, fleeing and...reproduction. Other behaviors, such as nonverbal communication like aggression and dominance, are born from this area of the brain. This part of the brain primarily consists of the upper brainstem and the hypothalamus (which should ring a bell from our earlier discussion about the body). As stated earlier, the hypothalamus plays a big role in fear regulation and recognition — as well as in modulating the ANS. *I want you to remember that last point.*

The next layer is the paleomammalian brain. It's wrapped around the first layer. It is primarily responsible for emotions and motivation. It also aids in learning and memory. Especially whenever you remember good or bad experiences. This layer contains the "limbic system." One of the main roles of this system is that it's the origin of value judgments that can sometimes, without our knowledge, affect our perception and — inevitably — our knowledge.

The last layer is the most complex layer. It's the most recent layer in terms of evolution. We call this layer the neomammalian cortex. In fact, this is the most important of the brain's neural architecture as it has allowed for the development of human language, abstract thought, and imagination. We're able to develop culture through the integration of this specific section of the brain. In fact, according to renowned neuroscientist Paul D. MacLean, this is the source of foresight, hindsight, and insight (Gould, 2003).

You might have to read this section one more time. I just want to make sure you understand the ideas and the language to get started. I promise — I'm going to connect it all in the next section. We'll be seeing how the brain's evolutionary hierarchy fits within the dysregulation of the autonomic system model (the one in the fear body chapter) and, more importantly, how this causes a feedback loop that distorts our minds and our perception of the world around us.

Let's take a step back (again). First, let's look at the earlier model I proposed about fear and the body. Here it is again:

Stressor -> Fear -> Amygdala -> Hypothalamus -> Sympathetic nervous system -> Chronic response -> Chronic fear -> Fear body

Something similar happens to our minds. In the same way that a chronic stressor is stored in our musculature and distorts our physical appearance (stress in the back, tight abdomens, psoas, etc.), so too do our minds get warped. We get into a state of perpetual tension and anxiety. Our thinking becomes narrow. We become hypersensitive to not only ourselves, but to everyone and even small criticisms. In fact, we sometimes even freeze and become paralyzed. Maybe we can't respond appropriately in the moment or even get ourselves out of bed in the morning.

In an ideal world, we would be able to process fear. We would see the scary stimulus or the emotion. This signal would be sent into the reptile brain, which would process the signal. Then, we could either activate the primitive system or we could understand it, see the biases, and gain better appreciation or understanding of what's going on.

Stressor -> Fear -> Reptile brain-> Paleomamallian -> Neomammalian -> Cognitive reappraisal and emotional regulation -> Homeostasis

The fear response would be modulated by the fact that it passes through multiple layers of the brain. Think of the layers as filters. Once the signal gets into the neomammalian region, it can get processed slowly and be analyzed. In fact, this most recent neomammalian cortex is where we hold reason. And that's wonderful. It helps to calm us down. It helps us see how absurd something anxiety-provoking is. It helps to lessen the fear and put it into place. Maybe we even crack a joke. The bottom line is this: the fear comes and goes away. It doesn't envelop us. We are able to move on and smile.

However, that's a rosy picture of life. Stress and fear are so prevalent in our modern world that, unfortunately, this regulation loop has been short circuited.

Chronic fear/Anxiety -> Reptile brain -> Amygdala -> Hypothalamus -> Sympathetic nervous system -> Fear mind

Chronic anxiety and worry give power to the most primitive and oldest part of the brain: the reptilian structure. This actually short-circuits our reasoning. It tints the way we look at the world and we start thinking like a reptile, focused on survival. We don't filter out our thoughts, biases, or emotions through the other two smarter and more evolved layers. Rather than a proactive and strategic manner, we stay stuck in a more primitive reactive manner of living

JUST TRY TO SURVIVE is what our evolutionary programming and our biology is telling our minds. This feedback loop gets more and more powerful as the stressors keep bombarding us. In fact, we get into the habit of a fearful mind. We are constantly stimulated, on edge. We are always frightened by even the smallest shadow, and we have difficulty in slowing down and understanding. As this constant reminder of danger is being etched into the mind, so too does the brain change. Neuroplasticity (the brain's ability to literally change, both functionally and even physically by our behaviors and thoughts) can make our brain less efficient. In fact, some studies have shown that constant stress and anxiety can change the size of certain regions of the brain (Pittenger & Duman, 2008).

But how do we fix this? Is our neurobiology so fixed that we can't even possibly go against this dysfunction? Are we a puppet to our evolution? Are we a puppet to biology?

Actually, no. It's not that hard. We can look at the wonderful work of neuroplasticity, and it tells us something. As Donald Hebb, a neuropsychologist said in 1948, "Neurons that fire together, wire together." And in that vein, if we do certain practices that help to fix this feedback loop (even just a little tweak here and there), it actually helps. It makes the system better. And it adds over time. In fact, the brains of people who work on this or make it a habit really do have different brains (Holzel 2010).

What is this magical way of fixing our emotional and, down the road, neurological issue of fear and anxiety?
One word: Mindfulness.

On Mindfulness

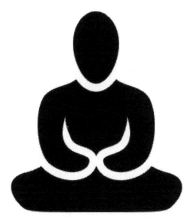

What is mindfulness? Well, I see it as the awareness of the day-to-day moments. You are conscious of the passage of time, but you aren't anchored to the past or yearning to the future. You are just existing. And you are savoring the moment. It sounds somewhat mystical. But really, it's the appreciation of the current moment and what feelings, sensations, and emotions are pulsating through your body.

When we discussed the fear mind and the chronic role of stress, we saw it as a dysregulation process — one whereby the mind and, subsequently, the brain maladapted to the environment. The constant tension of modernity short-circuits our fear response and causes us to use more primitive parts of our neurobiology. It's only meant for short-term survival, not long-term success.

In order to work on the fear mind, we need to practice habits and skills that bring us back to the homeostatic balance of the triune brain — but that's not all. We also need to straighten the connection and ability of the highest brain: the neomammalian context. Like a muscle, the techniques I present below require practice. They aren't easy as they are meant to push us sometimes into states of discomfort. And that's okay. We need to push through this.

Look at these exercises not as routines to calm yourself down or routines to slow down the world. Instead, I want you to consider these routines as habits and rituals that rebuild and rectify the neural circuits that were once dampened by the stress around you. I want you to consider meditation, or even mindfulness, akin to the way a sword needs to be continually sharpened to be useful.

OODA & BOODA Loop

I learned about the OODA loop while working on a Department of Defense project to secure their supercomputers. OODA was developed by a brilliant fighter pilot and military strategist named John Boyd.

This OODA loop is now used by business and sports strategists. As Wikipedia describes:

Boyd hypothesized that all intelligent organisms and organizations undergo a continuous cycle of interaction with their environment. Boyd breaks this cycle down to four interrelated and overlapping processes through which one cycles continuously:

Observation: the collection of data by means of the senses

Orientation: the analysis and synthesis of data to form one's current mental perspective

Decision: the determination of a course of action based on one's current mental perspective

Action: the physical playing-out of decisions

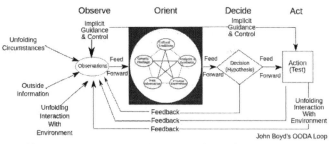

John Boyd's OODA Loop

Boyd's OODA has helped me to slow down during fast paced, intense, and important situations. It helps to reduce reactivity and promote proactive action.

It is a great framework but, I believe it is missing a step which can be helpful to anyone using it.
Breathe.

Breathe. Then observe, orient, decide, and act. Breathing puts us in a parasympathetic or relaxed state which allows for the most creative solution to appear.

I think John Boyd would dig the addition of the breathe step. He might even be okay with calling it the BOODA Loop.

———————

Similar to mindfulness, this is another technique that helps to bypass the anxiety circuit that fear causes. It helps us to get out of the "rut" or the loop that chronic fear creates. By doing this technique over and over again, especially in those moments of distress, we become better at it. To the point that it becomes even unconscious. We internalize the values of these exercises.

We want to get into a state where exercises that jolt us into the present become easier. And easier. So that we can harness this power of concentration without much effort.

Pausing to Take a Breath

Sometimes the most important thing we can do for ourselves is pause. What does it say on the side of a cereal box? *Contents may have settled.* In order for our mind to work efficiently in the long run, we need to allow it to settle. I wonder as I'm going through my day, "Have I taken the chance to settle?"

Try this the next time you're unsettled:
- Find a quiet place.
- Sit down, back straight up on a chair.
- Close your eyes.
- One inhalation through your nose.
- Exhale through your mouth.
- Observe your thoughts without judgement.

Postpone Worry

Here's one of the tactics I use: as soon as I realize I'm worrying about something out of my control, I will postpone it by distracting myself with a useful action. I'll go do something else and completely immerse myself in it.

Here's how to employ this tactic:

1. Choose an activity to engage your mind and body. It can even be simple like making some coffee, sweeping the floor, calling a friend to be of service to them.

2. Put your smartphone timer (or any other timer) on for 20 minutes.

3. Fully immerse yourself in the activity.

4. Observe at the end of the 20 minutes that you are probably less triggered by the worry.

If that doesn't work, repeat. At the end of the day, worry never gets anything done. As author and strategic consultant, Dan Zadra once said, "Worry is a miss-utilized form of the imagination."

Occam's Razor

Another technique to lessen stress in life is to use Occam's razor at every moment, which means to reduce, reduce, reduce. Do not add anything that may introduce more complexity into the equation. When we do this, again, we simplify life down to the bare bones and find that we have less drag. Essentially, we are aerodynamically more smooth, and there's fewer ripples that come out of life. In any single action or in a chain of actions, we can think, "What would make this the simplest?" Almost like cutting a hot knife through butter.

If you use a fork to cut through butter, the butter will spread all over the place. If you use a hot knife to cut through butter, then you are a lot smoother in the actions. The yogis refer to this when they talk about the drishti, a focal point that is employed during meditation or while holding a yoga pose. At any given moment, there is one point of awareness. That awareness and focal point allows you to cut through everything that's happening in life. At any given moment think, "What is my primary objective in this simple present moment?"

Conclusion

Let's look at Tim from the point of view of someone who has trained his mind.

Tim approaches the table. He recognizes that the game is on. He can feel his nerves starting to act up as his heart rate starts to increase. His palms feel sweaty. In fact, he feels a little uneasy. But it's okay, he tells himself. He recognizes that he has awareness about his thoughts. He understands that there is a loop of catastrophizing the worst-case scenario playing in his mind, over and over again. He understands that the bright lights, the allure of alcohol and seduction, and even the fast-paced nature of the game are short-circuiting his brain.

With this appreciation of his thinking, Tim sees the absurdity of his thoughts. He pauses to take a breath. He recognizes all the reactions that his body is emanating as just responses from his sympathetic system. He uses the BOODA Loop to slow down the world around him and returns his focus to the present poker hand. And gradually things get better. Tim knows that he needs to practice this type of thinking more often in order to internalize the values and make good habits.

At the end of the day, our perceptions shape our brains, and our brains shape our perceptions. It's a two-way street. It's on us to take responsibility for how we look at the world and how we condition both our bodies and our minds to react. Stress and anxiety will always exist. But our reactions, our outlooks, our mindsets or the way we observe these events can really influence the way they affect us. This in turn also regulates our ANS and, therefore, our sympathetic and parasympathetic behaviors.

In this chapter, we discussed the importance of the "fear mind," or a model of how anxiety and chronic stress can short-circuit our minds. We used the triune brain as a model of how evolution has sculpted the brain and how the stressors of our modern society can bypass the regulatory systems in the brain. This in turn causes so many problems — constant worry, lack of focus, tension, a narrower mind, and paranoia.

Summary

- The brain is composed of multiple layers of complexity that follow evolution (triune brain).
- Chronic stress and anxiety can affect the communication between parts of the brain.
- We can use mindfulness and other techniques to help strengthen good communication between various layers of the brain to affect the mind.

Conclusion

At the end of the day, stressful events are inevitable. Stress is a part of our lives and the decisions we make. We can either choose to let it wash over us and let it dominate our lives, or we can learn, understand, and grow from it., And our nervous system is key to this decision, particularly the balance between our sympathetic (on/go) and parasympathetic (off/slow) systems. We see that stress isn't just the tension we feel before getting an unexpected message from our boss or the anxiety we have when driving. No, it's much more than that. It's also a concoction of various chemicals that surge through our body, our habits and the tools we use to address it.

Chapter 1 was an introduction to the nervous system and its role with stress. The nervous system has a variety of sub-systems, but we focused on the sympathetic and parasympathetic dichotomy and how this division helps to modulate our stress and fear response. You learned some basics about the ANS and the different subsystems including the vagus nerve and the fight-flight response.

In chapter 2, you saw that the way we breathe can affect the ANS. The way we inhale oxygen and both the intensity and depth of these inhalations can modulate the ANS. Breathing techniques can stimulate our vagus nerve, hence causing a higher relaxation response. I hope that I was able to impart to you a few techniques, some of which I do on a daily basis, to help slow your breathing and get more into a relaxed state.

In chapter 3, we had a discussion about the body. This isn't just the typical discussion on how to fix your posture or the way you sit down to talk. No, I hope it was a wakeup call that the way you hold your body in space and the way your mind follows is a unique relationship. Our physicality can shape the way we perceive the world and can make us feel more confident. In contrast, chronic stress distorts and disfigures our posture. We hold stress in our pelvic and abdominal region, especially in the psoas, causing tension in the lower back. I call this the "fear body," and I think it helps to explain why we store stress in these regions. We also discussed a few techniques, including the constructive rest posture, to open up the lower back and relieve some of the tension and stress that we've built up that has been stored in our muscles.

Chapter 4 was an introduction to the triune brain and how both neuroanatomy and mindfulness can shape the brain's response to stress. You saw that the various layers each have a specific function and work in concert with one another. But with chronic stress and anxiety, the communication between the most primitive and most advanced sections are disrupted, causing the "freeze" response and a variety of other maladaptive thoughts. And so the very structure of the brain helped to create the narrow view of the world that limits us. It could be that this miscommunication plays a key role in how we perceive stress and how we are able to cope with it. We also discussed the importance of mindfulness and other techniques to get out of "fear mind."

I hope this short book has inspired you and piqued your interest in nervous system hacking. This is just the beginning of our quest for a healthier mind and healthier body, less stress and more success. In the next book in the Hacking Your Nervous System series, we will be exploring nutrition as a way to reprogram the nervous system and a revolutionary body practice to discharge stress. I look forward to hearing from you and joining your path towards a more successful and less stressful life.

Appendix: From The Blog

Why is Barry White's voice so appealing?

Barry White's voice has all of the qualities normally associated with good poetry, a term called 'prosody,' which in linguistics, refers to units of speech and rhythm, tone, form, intonation, and so forth. When you hear something aurally pleasing, it is typically also prosodic.

Prosodic speech has the qualities of safety and connectedness, groundedness and openness, and *presence*.

When someone speaks in this way, we're subconsciously sizing them up for their reproductive potential, which means we're looking for a host of other great qualities in mate-seeking behavior. The process of 'sizing-up for reproductive potential' is something that everybody does in some form or another, and is an evolutionary protective measure that helped the human species over time. We seek security, safety, social cohesion, and compatibility. It's not hard to listen to a single Barry White track and understand why people love the sound of his voice — it has all of these characteristics.

These characteristics are symptomatic of an autonomic nervous system that is in the ventral-vagal-state. Ventral-vagal just means a state of being closely related to either secure and grounded. It stems from Polyvagal theory, developed by Dr. Stephen Porges. In Polyvagal theory, socio-emotional interaction and response are dictated by the firing patterns of the autonomic nervous system, and they can either be secure or insecure.

'Insecure' in these terms doesn't mean petty or lacking confidence — it means overburdened by stress. 'Secure' on the other hand doesn't (always) mean having the confidence and sex appeal of Barry White, but rather, it means being collected and extremely chilled out.

A nervous system like Barry's is in the ventral-vagal parasympathetic state. That means he's:
- More likely than not to be resistant to infection
- Have a strong immune response, greater levels of oxytocin (a neuromodulator for social bonds)
- Deeper breath
- Longer intervals of rest and recuperation
- Much better circulation to the non-vital organs such as the digestive and reproductive systems.

These are also the qualities we inadvertently seek in others as an evolutionary mechanism to ensure higher reproductive success.

So there you have it — it's not just you — we *all* can't get enough of Barry White's voice, baby.

The Human Blue Screen of Death...

A couple of decades ago in the Ötztal Alps of southern Austria, two German tourists stumbled upon one of the best-preserved human specimens from around 3300 BCE. He was frozen into a mountain. Forensic and biological anthropologists/archaeologists named him Ötzi and still dispute the cause of his death, but I want to pose a conditional hypothesis. Contingent upon Ötzi's death being a struggle-and-a-wane, I'm going to suggest that there was a period of time during which he entered a 'frozen' state as his body began shutting down.

The takeaway here is that he fought, sustained trauma, and had nowhere else to go, so he froze at first neurologically, thanks to the longstanding evolutionary mechanism that is the Dorsal Vagal Parasympathetic Nervous System, and then he froze literally, thanks to...the alps.

The human Nervous System sometimes enters into a frozen state--it's called the Dorsal Vagal Parasympathetic Nervous System (DVS), which is part of the Autonomic Nervous System (ANS). The DVS is one of the oldest parts evolved into our ANSs, and it serves to protect in moments where we can neither dodge a situation or fight through it. The alternative to fight-or-flight reaction is activation of the DVS. It immobilizes the individual, acting as a sort of emergency break in the human body. 'Human blue screen of death' aptly describes the sum total of the effects of the freeze-response.

Picture giving a public speech and choking because you're unable to perform in that moment, or sitting down to take a test and immediately feeling like you forgot everything you studied. Feeling overwhelmed happens not just on the mental level--it happens physiologically, too. That's why it's hard to move when it hits.

All of this happens because the nervous system goes into overdrive in order to protect the body from potential physical harm. It's meant for life-threatening moments, but the bio/physiological mechanism has carried over into modern living.

When we respond to events we can't dodge or plow through, and go frozen, we also experience a bunch of physiological effects which are designed to help conserve energy in the event that the worst-case scenario happens (death or being attacked): decreased heart rate, a slowed rate of respiration, shock and disassociation, higher threshold for pain (the body produces opioids that help to numb it), hyper-distracted hypervigilance, and a frozen facial expression that comes off as defensive. It's hard to maintain eye contact because the body is distracting itself from the situation at hand. If we're privileged enough to be able to speak in this state, it sure doesn't sound as aurally pleasing as Barry White. The voice shakes, takes on a higher pitch than what is normal for an individual, and sounds threatened or reactive.

When we're frozen, we're disconnected, barely breathing, sitting very still, spinning internally, unavailable to connect and communicate effectively, and incapable of doing our jobs well, if at all.

People cope to decompress and phase stress out with a variety of strategies, some good, some bad-- self-care routines, going to yoga, aggressively cleaning, participating in extreme sports for a hit of adrenaline; alcohol, smoking weed, eating junk food; without calculation, engaging in risky behavior like sleeping around, 'getting into trouble,' spending time with destructive or toxic people, self-destructing without realizing it, or self-harming. These are *all distractions.*

Common self-harming behaviors associated with not managing the freeze-response include addiction, cutting, eating disorders (*including* binge eating), and actively practicig low self-esteem. We can easily slip into depression when we're doing these things that we think are helping, but are actually harming. It's a positive feedback loop--the more that stress goes in, it compounds the coping mechanisms into habit, and this continues until an individual is thoroughly destabilized and desperately needs help.

The song 'Let it Go' from the movie Frozen comes to mind. Truth be told, there's really only one verse that applies with respect to this discussion:

It's time to see what I can do
To test the limits and break through
No right, no wrong, no rules for me,
I'm free!

When we recognize that we're freezing up and take steps to preemptively thaw ourselves out, through breath and strategic relaxation practices, some pretty radical things happen.

Foremost, and what is commonly associated with consuming hallucinogenic material, the meditation brings a loss of self, or a reduction in the importance of ego in one's everyday cognition. Next, which doesn't suck, people report having mind-blowing sex without really doing anything differently in terms of spicing it up. Finally, a sensation of balance, well-being, and 'doing it right' comes in and opens one up to being happy. Not the superficial 'happy' that the Pharrell song commands us to feel, but the 'happy' that follows feeling totally secure in one's body, thoughts, and life.

Breathing and Brain Waves

Breathing has long been used by yogis and kung fu artists to enhance cognitive function and modulate emotions such as fear.

A recent study in *The Journal of Neuroscience* discusses the ability of breathing to entrain mood and focus.

"Nasal Respiration Entrains Human Limbic Oscillations and Modulates Cognitive Function" by Zelano et al.

Zelano notes:

"If you are in a panic state, your breathing rhythm becomes faster. As a result you'll spend proportionally more time inhaling than when in a calm state. Thus, our body's innate response to fear, with faster breathing, could have a positive impact

on brain function and result in faster response times

to dangerous stimuli in the environment."

"When you inhale, you are in a sense synchronizing

brain oscillations across the limbic network."

The limbic system handles emotional processing in the brain. "Going limbic" means to be overwhelmed by emotion and to lose rational processing.

Here's a couple takeaways:

- Breathe through the nose.
- Keep a smooth rhythm of breath to calm the brain.

Breath is like the timing belt of your body. If you feel like you're "off," or out of whack, bring the attention to the rhythm of breath. Smooth inhale, smooth exhale.

3 Reasons to Blow Your Nose Before Sex

There are three critical reasons you should blow your nose before sex.

The first reason you need to blow your nose before sex is to lessen histamine response. Histamine is what happens when there's an allergen in your body. Histamine gets the body all excited. All of a sudden, the body starts over reacting to the pollen and you start unconsciously sneezing. That same histamine response brings the body into the sympathetic mode, gets a bunch of nerves engaged, pumps cortisol and adrenaline - the neurotransmitters of fight-flight, and that gets you closer to ejaculation and orgasm. If you're in an excited/allergic state, then you're not going to get a good erection or may have a hard time moistening the vagina because when cortisol and adrenaline is pumping through the body and you're in a fight-flight mode. If you do get a good erection, you will be apt to ejaculate faster because the body is in a fight-flight state. It's not in a fully relaxed state.

The second one is that when we breathe through the nose, it increases nitric oxide in the bloodstream. Nitric oxide is the same thing that the little blue pill works on to increase vasodilation. Vasodilation opens the veins in the body so the blood can pump more forcefully throughout the body. This is critical for getting an erection or for engorgement of the vagina. You need to breathe through the nose to get the blood flowing.

The third reason you should breathe through the nose is because it stimulates the parasympathetic nervous system and the vagus nerve. The vagus nerve is responsible for calming the body, for rest, digest, and nest. Nest means have sex. The vagus nerve connects from the brain to the pelvic region to stimulate time for relaxation and play. If you want to be relaxed and have sex last a long time, the vagus nerve needs to be working well. When you orgasm, that's caused by the opposite nerve called the visceral nerve. The visceral chain ganglia is what gets the body all excited. In order for you to have a long session of sex, inhale through the nose to stimulate the vagus nerve. If you want even more calming energy, as you exhale, make any sound you body feels like making. A grunt, a groan, a moan. The more excited you get the louder the sound. This is called resistance breathing which is covered in the breathing chapter.

One reason to bring your girlfriend flowers and chocolate is that they stimulate the histamine receptors which can promote the needed sympathetic response necessary for orgasm.

As a side, as you get closer to orgasm and want to climax, breathe deep and hard through the mouth.

Keep this in mind the next time you go to have sex and give that a try.
Go blow your nose. Make sure both nostrils are fully open. If you start to get too excited, take longer, slower, and deeper breaths through the nose.

Citations and References

Chapter 1: Intro to ANS

Ebrecht, Marcel et al. "Perceived Stress and Cortisol Levels Predict Speed of Wound Healing in Healthy Male Adults." *Psychoneuroendocrinology* 29.6 (2004): 798–809. Web.

Las Vegas image. Vecteezy.com

Beauchaine, Theodore. "Vagal tone, development, and Gray's motivational theory: Toward an integrated model of autonomic nervous system functioning in psychopathology" *Development and Psychopathology,* **13** (2001), 183–214.

Field, Tiffany, and Miguel Diego. "Vagal Activity, Early Growth and Emotional Development." *Infant Behavior and Development* 31.3 (2008): 361-73. *PubMed*. Web. 19 Nov. 2016.

Moore, Ginger A. "Parent Conflict Predicts Infants' Vagal Regulation in Social Interaction." *Dev Psychopathol Development and Psychopathology* 22.01 (2010): 23. *PubMed*. Web. 19 Nov. 2016.

Jones, Robin M., Anthony P. Buhr, Edward G. Conture, Victoria Tumanova, Tedra A. Walden, and

Stephen W. Porges. "Autonomic Nervous System Activity of Preschool-age Children Who Stutter." *Journal of Fluency Disorders* 41 (2014): 12-31. *PubMed*. Web. 19 Nov. 2016.

Waldburger, Jean-Marc, and Gary S. Firestein. "Regulation of Peripheral Inflammation by the Central Nervous System." *Current Rheumatology Reports* 12.5 (2010): 370-78. *Pubmed*. Web. 20 Nov. 2016.

Haley, Robert W., Elizabeth Charuvastra, William E. Shell, David M. Buhner, W. Wesley Marshall, Melanie M. Biggs, Steve C. Hopkins, Gil I. Wolfe, and Steven Vernino. "Cholinergic Autonomic Dysfunction in Veterans With Gulf War Illness." *JAMA Neurology*70.2 (2013): 191. Web. 20 Nov. 2016.

Pamenter, Matthew E., and Frank L. Powell. "Time Domains of the Hypoxic Ventilatory Response and Their Molecular Basis." *Comprehensive Physiology* (2016): 1345-385. Web. 20 Nov. 2016.

Chapter 2: Breath
Intro

Moore, Monique, David Brown, Nisha Money, and Mark Bates. "Mind-body Techniques for Regulating the Autonomic Nervous System." Http://www.dcoe.mil/. Defense Centers of Excellence for Psychological Health & Traumatic Brain Injury, n.d. Web. 18 Dec. 2016.

Deep Breathing

Bernardi, Luciano, Alessandra Gabutti, Cesare Porta, and Lucia Spicuzza. "Slow Breathing Reduces

Chemoreflex Response to Hypoxia and Hypercapnia, and Increases Baroreflex Sensitivity." Journal of Hypertension 19.12 (2001): 2221-229. Web. 20 Dec. 2016.

Jerath, Ravinder, John W. Edry, Vernon A. Barnes, and Vandna Jerath. "Physiology of Long Pranayamic Breathing: Neural Respiratory Elements May Provide a Mechanism That Explains How Slow Deep Breathing Shifts the Autonomic Nervous System." Medical Hypotheses 67.3 (2006): 566-71. Web. 20 Dec. 2016.

Lawenda, M.D. Brian D. "Powerful Relaxation Technique: 4-7-8 Breathing." Integrative Oncology Essentials. N.p., 13 Jan. 2016. Web. 20 Dec. 2016.

Pramanik, Tapas, Hari Om Sharma, Suchita Mishra, Anurag Mishra, Rajesh Prajapati, and Smriti Singh. "Immediate Effect of Slow Pace Bhastrika Pranayama on Blood Pressure and Heart Rate." The Journal of Alternative and Complementary Medicine 15.3 (2009): 293-95. Web. 20 Dec. 2016.

Sinha, Anant Narayan. "Assessment of the Effects of Pranayama/Alternate Nostril Breathing on the Parasympathetic Nervous System in Young Adults." Journal Of Clinical And Diagnostic Research (2013): n. pag. Web. 20 Dec. 2016.

Fear Breathing

Albrecht, E., E. Sillanpaa, S. Karrasch, A. C. Alves, V. Codd, I. Hovatta, J. L. Buxton, C. P. Nelson, L. Broer, S. Hagg, M. Mangino, G. Willemsen, I. Surakka, M. A. R. Ferreira, N. Amin, B. A. Oostra, H. M.

Backmand, M. Peltonen, S. Sarna, T. Rantanen, S. Sipila, T. Korhonen, P. A. F. Madden, C. Gieger, R. A. Jorres, J. Heinrich, J. Behr, R. M. Huber, A. Peters, K. Strauch, H. E. Wichmann, M. Waldenberger, A. I. F. Blakemore, E. J. C. De Geus, D. R. Nyholt, A. K. Henders, P. L. Piirila, A. Rissanen, P. K. E. Magnusson, A. Vinuela, K. H. Pietilainen, N. G. Martin, N. L. Pedersen, D. I. Boomsma, T. D. Spector, C. M. Van Duijn, J. Kaprio, N. J. Samani, M.-R. Jarvelin, and H. Schulz. "Telomere Length in Circulating Leukocytes Is Associated with Lung Function and Disease." European Respiratory Journal 43.4 (2013): 983-92. Pubmed. Web. 17 Dec. 2016.

Fried, Robert. The Breath Connection: How to Reduce Psychosomatic and Stress-related Disorders with Easy-to-do Breathing Exercises. New York: Insight, 1990. Print.

Meerman, R., and A. J. Brown. "When Somebody Loses Weight, Where Does the Fat Go?"BMJ 349.Dec16 13 (2014): n. pag. Web.

Tolentino, Elen De Souza, Luiz Eduardo Montenegro Chinellato, and Olinda Tarzia. "Saliva and Tongue Coating PH before and after Use of Mouthwashes and Relationship with Parameters of Halitosis." Journal of Applied Oral Science 19.2 (2011): 90-94. Web. 20 Dec. 2016.

University of New South Wales. "When you lose weight, where does the fat go? Most of the mass is breathed out as carbon dioxide, study shows." ScienceDaily. ScienceDaily, 16 December 2014.

<www.sciencedaily.com/releases/2014/12/1412162
12047.htm>.

Exercises

https://pixabay.com/en/meditation-girl-temple-quiet-972472/
https://pixabay.com/en/diver-diving-underwater-adventure-311634/
https://pixabay.com/en/parachuting-parachute-glide-falling-1781587/

https://pixabay.com/en/target-sniper-bullseye-aim-aiming-41357/
https://pixabay.com/en/running-runner-long-distance-573762/

Bernadi, Luciano et al. "Effect of rosary prayer and yoga mantras on autonomic cardiovascular rhythms: comparative study." BMJ. 2001 Dec 22; 323(7327): 1446–1449.

Martarelli, Daniele, Mario Cocchioni, Stefania Scuri, and Pierluigi Pompei. "Diaphragmatic Breathing Reduces Exercise-Induced Oxidative Stress." Evidence-Based Complementary and Alternative Medicine 2011 (2011): 1-10. Web. 21 Dec. 2016.

Milton, S. "Go Ahead, Vent Your Spleen!" Journal of Experimental Biology 207.3 (2004): 390. Web. 21 Dec. 2016.

"Why Does Blood Become More Acidic When Carbon Dioxide Increases?"LIVESTRONG.COM. Leaf Group, 19 Feb. 2014. Web. 20 Dec. 2016.

Schagatay, Erika, Matt X. Richardson, and Angelica Lodin-Sundström. "Size Matters: Spleen and Lung Volumes Predict Performance in Human Apneic Divers." Frontiers in Physiology 3 (2012): n. pag. Web. 22 Dec. 2016.

"SEALFIT - Slow Is Smooth...Smooth Is Fast." Navy SEALs. N.p., 7–7 Feb. 2014. Web. 23 Dec. 2016.

Telles, S., R. Nagarathna, and HR Nagendra. "Breathing through a Particular Nostril Can Alter Metabolism and Autonomic Activities." Indian Journal of Physiology and Pharmacology(1994): n. pag. Pubmed. Web. 20 Dec. 2016.

Vickhoff, Bjorn, Helge Malmgren, Gunnar Nyberg, Seth-Reino Ekstrom, Mathias Engwall, Johan Snygg, Michael Nilsson, Rebecka Jornsten, and Rickard Astrom. "Music Structure Determines Heart Rate Variability of Singers." Frontiers in Psychology 4 (2013): n. pag. Web. 21 Dec. 2016.

Conclusion
Hanh, Thich Nhat. "Stepping into Freedom Quotes." Goodreads.com. N.p., n.d. Web. 22 Dec. 2016.

Chapter 3: Body
Intro

https://jhunwa.blogspot.com/2012/01/old-school-windows-game-skifree.html

Mehrabian, A., and S. R. Ferris. "Inference of Attitudes from Nonverbal Communication in Two Channels." Journal of Consulting Psychology 31.3 (1967): 248–252. Print.

Fear Body

https://morguefile.com/search/morguefile/3/fear/pop

https://morguefile.com/search/morguefile/10/scary/pop

https://pixabay.com/en/girl-woman-portrait-character-1660891/

https://en.wikipedia.org/wiki/File:Psoas_major_muscle11.png

https://en.wikipedia.org/wiki/File:Anterior_Hip_Muscles_2.PNG

Berceli, PhD, David, and MD Scaer Robert. Shake It Off Naturally: Reduce Stress, Anxiety, and Tension with. CreateSpace Independent Publishing Platform, 2015. Print.

Borgomaneri, Sara et al. "Seeing Fearful Body Language Rapidly Freezes the Observer's Motor Cortex." Cortex; a Journal Devoted to the Study of the Nervous System and Behavior 65 (2015): 232–245. Web.

Carney, Dana R., Amy J. C. Cuddy, and Andy J. Yap. "Power Posing: Brief Nonverbal Displays Affect Neuroendocrine Levels and Risk Tolerance."

Psychological Science 21.10 (2010): 1363–1368. Web.

---. "Review and Summary of Research on the Embodied Effects of Expansive (vs. Contractive) Nonverbal Displays." Psychological Science 26.5 (2015): 657–663. Web.

Cuddy, Amy J. C. et al. "Preparatory Power Posing Affects Nonverbal Presence and Job Interview Performance." The Journal of Applied Psychology 100.4 (2015): 1286–1295. Web.

de Gelder, Beatrice. "Towards the Neurobiology of Emotional Body Language." Nature Reviews Neuroscience 7.3 (2006): 242–249. Web. 31 Dec. 2016.

Grèzes, J., S. Pichon, and B. de Gelder. "Perceiving Fear in Dynamic Body Expressions." NeuroImage 35.2 (2007): 959–967. Web. 31 Dec. 2016.

Amy Cuddy and Power Poses
http://www.fccorange.com/multimedia-archive/2014_04_20/

Cuddy, Amy. Presence: Bringing Your Boldest Self to Your Biggest Challenges. First Edition: December 2015 edition. New York: Little, Brown and Company, 2015. Print.

Exercises
https://pixabay.com/en/football-game-referee-players-youth-1647128/

"5 Power Poses You Should Start Using at Work Now." Levo League. N.p., 23 Jan. 2014. Web. 7 Jan. 2017.

"Body Language Hacks: Be Confident and Reduce Stress in 2 Minutes." James Clear. N.p., 25–25 July 2013. Web. 7 Jan. 2017.

"Iliopsoas Release: Constructive Rest Position." CoreWalking. N.p., 3–3 Aug. 2011. Web. 7 Jan. 2017.

"Power Up With These 5 Poses." N.p., n.d. Web. 7 Jan. 2017.

Chapter 4: Mind
Intro
https://pixabay.com/en/the-gaps-picture-explore-prayer-1525191/
Triune Brain

Baars, Bernard J., and Nicole M. Gage. "Chapter 13 - Emotion." Cognition, Brain, and Consciousness (Second Edition). London: Academic Press, 2010. 420–442. Web. 15 Jan. 2017.

Gould, Jay E. "Triune Brain Concept." (n.d.): n. pag. Http://uwf.edu/jgould. 10 Sept. 2003. Web. 14 Jan. 2017.

Holden, C. "Paul MacLean and the Triune Brain." Science (New York, N.Y.) 204.4397 (1979): 1066–1068. Print.

Duboc, Bruno. "THE BRAIN FROM TOP TO BOTTOM." THE BRAIN FROM TOP TO BOTTOM. McGill University, n.d. Web. 14 Jan. 2017.

Fear Mind

Zeidan, Fadel et al. "Neural Correlates of Mindfulness Meditation-Related Anxiety Relief." Social Cognitive and Affective Neuroscience 9.6 (2014): 751–759. Web.

"How to Grow the Good in Your Brain." Greater Good. N.p., n.d. Web. 12 Jan. 2017.

Kolassa, Iris-Tatjana, and Thomas Elbert. "Structural and Functional Neuroplasticity in Relation to Traumatic Stress." Current Directions in Psychological Science 16.6 (2007): 321–325. Web. 12 Jan. 2017.

PhD, Ruth Baer, ed. Assessing Mindfulness and Acceptance Processes in Clients: Illuminating the Theory and Practice of Change. 1 edition. Oakland, CA: Context Press, 2010. Print.

Pittenger, Christopher, and Ronald S. Duman. "Stress, Depression, and Neuroplasticity: A Convergence of Mechanisms." Neuropsychopharmacology 33.1 (2007): 88–109. Web. 12 Jan. 2017.

Holzel, Britta et al. "Stress reduction correlates with structural changes in the amygdala." Soc Cogn Affect Neurosci. 2010 Mar;5(1):11-7. doi: 10.1093/scan/nsp034. Epub 2009 Sep 23.

Exercises

https://upload.wikimedia.org/wikipedia/commons/3/3a/OODA.Boyd.svg

"Boyd's O.O.D.A Loop and How We Use It." Tactical Response. N.p., n.d. Web. 14 Jan. 2017.

Testimonials For My Corporate & Personal Training Classes

The techniques learned were extremely

effective at helping me recenter and refocus before starting my next task. The staff who participated were very grateful. They expressed afterward how much they appreciated the workshop and the agency focusing on 'their self-care.' They are looking forward to the next workshop!
— Jessica MacLeod, MSW, Director of Social Services, Thrive DC

Our time with Rob was such a relaxing

experience...I fell asleep.
— Anonymous

I dealt with extreme stress at the end of

2016 / early 2017 and I wish I had known how to better manage the physical aspects of it. Would love to learn more- about the tremors, I always thought they were a sign of muscle weakness or lack of control.
— Anonymous

I learned how to escape my stressful

thoughts and worries and to just be in the moment. I haven't felt that relaxed in a long time.
— K. Herhold

I really enjoyed that experience. I always

forget the importance of stepping back, listening to the body, so that was greatly appreciated. Thank you! Favorite part was the tremoring—so weird but very interesting!
— Jenna

I haven't felt this connected to my body in

a long time. I've had anxiety for years and this workshop taught me some very useful tools to handle it moving forward.
— C.G., a Broadcast News Anchor

This workshop melted away my stress

during a time of anxiety and stress.
— S. Philibotte

Want The Next Level?
Get my favorite tips and take the training to the
next level at: http://robhartman.co

May I Ask A Favor?
I would really appreciate it if you would post a short review of this book on Amazon. Good or bad, just make it honest to help others in their choice.

Thank You!

Made in the USA
Columbia, SC
30 April 2018